CHRONIC WASTING DISEASES

DEER,TRANSMISSIBLE SPONGIFORM ENCEPHALOPATHY

BY

JAKE.B.BUSH

Table of Contents

Chapter 1

INTRODUCTION

Overview of Chronic Wasting Diseases (CWD)

Chronic Wasting Disease (CWD) is a progressive and fatal neurological disorder primarily affecting members of the deer family, including deer, elk, and moose. It belongs to a group of diseases known as Transmissible Spongiform Encephalopathies (TSEs), characterized by abnormal protein folding leading to the accumulation of prions in the brain.

CWD has garnered increasing attention due to its impact on wildlife populations and concerns about potential transmission to other species, including humans. The disease is distinguished by its slow incubation period and the distinct spongy degeneration of the brain, resulting in behavioral changes, weight loss, and eventual death.

Understanding the epidemiology, causative agents (prions), and effective management strategies are crucial in addressing the challenges posed by CWD. Ongoing research aims to unravel the complexities of the disease, with a focus on preventing further spread and mitigating its ecological and economic consequences.

Significance in Deer Populations

Chronic Wasting Disease (CWD) holds considerable significance within deer populations, influencing both the individual animals and the broader ecological landscape. As a contagious and fatal neurodegenerative disorder, CWD poses a threat to the health and sustainability of deer herds.

1. Population Dynamics: CWD can lead to a decline in deer populations over time. Infected individuals often exhibit changes in behavior, decreased reproductive success, and increased

mortality, impacting the overall population structure.

2. Ecological Balance: Deer play a crucial role in maintaining ecological balance through their influence on vegetation and as prey for predators. The disruption caused by CWD can have cascading effects on the entire ecosystem, affecting plant communities and predator-prey relationships.

3. Economic Implications: Deer populations are of economic importance, contributing to wildlife-related industries such as hunting and ecotourism. The presence of CWD can result in decreased hunting opportunities, affecting both recreational and economic aspects associated with deer management.

4. Challenges for Conservation: The spread of CWD presents a challenge for conservation efforts, requiring effective strategies to monitor, manage, and mitigate its impact on deer populations. Conservationists and wildlife managers face the task of balancing population

control measures with the preservation of healthy ecosystems.

Understanding the significance of CWD in deer populations is crucial for implementing proactive measures to control its spread, protect biodiversity, and sustain the ecological integrity of deer-inhabited regions.

Chapter 2

Understanding Transmissible Spongiform Encephalopathy (TSE)

Transmissible Spongiform Encephalopathy (TSE) represents a group of rare and fatal neurodegenerative disorders that affect the central nervous system. These diseases are characterized by the accumulation of misfolded prion proteins, leading to distinctive spongy changes in brain tissue.

1. Nature and Characteristics: TSEs, including Chronic Wasting Disease (CWD), share common features such as a long incubation period and the progressive degeneration of neurological tissues. The term "spongiform" refers to the sponge-like appearance of affected brain tissue under microscopic examination.

2. Prions: Culprit in TSE: The primary causative agents of TSEs are abnormal prion proteins. Prions are misfolded versions of a normal

cellular protein that can induce the misfolding of their healthy counterparts. This aberrant protein folding process leads to the formation of insoluble aggregates, damaging neural tissue.

3. Mechanisms of Transmission: TSEs can be transmitted horizontally through direct contact or exposure to contaminated materials, as well as vertically from parent to offspring. Prions are exceptionally resistant to standard sterilization methods, complicating efforts to control their spread.

4. Variety of TSEs: TSEs manifest in different forms across species, including Creutzfeldt-Jakob Disease (CJD) in humans, Bovine Spongiform Encephalopathy (BSE) in cattle, and Scrapie in sheep. Each variation exhibits unique characteristics but shares the commonality of prion-induced neurodegeneration.

Understanding TSEs is fundamental for addressing the complexities associated with diseases like CWD. Research continues to delve into the intricate mechanisms of prion propagation, aiding in the development of diagnostic methods, preventive measures, and potential treatments for these challenging neurological disorders.

Nature and Characteristics of TSE

Transmissible Spongiform Encephalopathy (TSE) is a group of neurodegenerative diseases characterized by distinct pathological changes in the brain tissue. The nature and characteristics of TSE contribute to the unique and challenging aspects of these disorders.

1. Long Incubation Period: TSEs are notable for their unusually long incubation periods, during which infected individuals may show no outward signs of the disease. This prolonged latency makes it challenging to detect and control the spread of TSEs in affected populations.

2. Prion-Induced Misfolding: At the core of TSE pathology is the abnormal folding of prion proteins. Normally present in a harmless form,

these proteins undergo a structural transformation, adopting a misfolded conformation. The accumulation of these misfolded prions in the brain leads to neuronal damage and the characteristic spongiform appearance.

3. Spongiform Changes in Brain Tissue: Upon microscopic examination, affected brain tissue reveals sponge-like holes and vacuoles, a hallmark feature of TSEs. These structural alterations result from the destruction of neurons and the accumulation of abnormal prion proteins, causing a progressive and irreversible deterioration of neurological function.

4. Variability Across Species: While TSEs share common features, variations exist among species. For instance, Bovine Spongiform Encephalopathy (BSE) in cattle, Scrapie in sheep, and Chronic Wasting Disease (CWD) in deer exhibit species-specific characteristics. Understanding these variations is crucial for tailored diagnostic approaches and control strategies.

5. Resistance to Standard Sterilization Methods: Prions responsible for TSEs display remarkable resistance to conventional sterilization methods. This resistance contributes to the persistence of prions in the environment and complicates efforts to eliminate or reduce their transmission.

Comprehending the nature and characteristics of TSEs is essential for developing effective diagnostic tools, preventive measures, and management strategies. Ongoing research aims to unravel the intricate details of prion biology, providing insights into the mechanisms of disease progression and potential avenues for intervention.

Mechanisms of Transmission in Transmissible Spongiform Encephalopathy (TSE)

Transmissible Spongiform Encephalopathies (TSEs) are characterized by their unique modes of transmission, contributing to the challenges in controlling and preventing the spread of these neurodegenerative diseases.

1. Direct Contact and Horizontal Transmission: TSEs can be transmitted horizontally through direct contact between infected and susceptible individuals. This can occur through shared environments, bodily fluids, or contact with contaminated surfaces. Horizontal transmission is a significant factor in the spread of TSEs within animal populations.

2. Ingestion of Contaminated Material: The ingestion of contaminated material, such as prion-infected tissues or environmental reservoirs containing prions, is a common route of transmission. This mechanism is particularly relevant in herbivorous species like deer, where

exposure to contaminated vegetation or soil plays a crucial role in disease transmission.

3. Vertical Transmission: In some cases, TSEs can be transmitted vertically from an infected parent to its offspring. This mode of transmission occurs during gestation or through the consumption of infected milk. Understanding vertical transmission is essential for comprehending the persistence of TSEs within populations over successive generations.

4. Environmental Persistence: Prions, the infectious agents in TSEs, exhibit remarkable resistance to degradation. This resilience allows them to persist in the environment for extended periods, contributing to the ongoing transmission of TSEs even in areas where infected individuals may no longer be present.

5. Reservoirs and Indirect Transmission: TSEs can be maintained in the environment through reservoirs of infectious prions. Indirect transmission occurs when susceptible individuals come into contact with these reservoirs, leading to new infections. This

aspect adds complexity to efforts aimed at preventing TSE transmission.

Chapter 3

Chronic Wasting Diseases in Deer

Chronic Wasting Disease (CWD) poses a significant threat to deer populations, presenting unique challenges to wildlife management and conservation efforts.

- Species Affected: CWD affects various species within the deer family, including white-tailed deer, mule deer, elk, and moose. The susceptibility of multiple species contributes to the complexity of understanding and controlling the disease.

- Geographical Distribution: CWD has demonstrated a growing geographical distribution, with reported cases in North America, South Korea, and parts of Europe. The widespread nature of the disease underscores the need for coordinated efforts in monitoring, prevention, and control on a global scale.

- Clinical Symptoms in Deer: Infected deer exhibit distinct clinical symptoms, including progressive weight loss, altered behavior, excessive salivation, and physical debilitation. These signs reflect the neurodegenerative nature of the disease, with misfolded prion proteins accumulating in the brain, leading to severe neurological damage and ultimately death.

CWD represents a multifaceted challenge, impacting the health of deer populations and raising concerns about potential transmission to other species, including humans. Efforts to manage and mitigate the impact of CWD involve a comprehensive understanding of its epidemiology, causative agents, and strategies for surveillance and control. Wildlife authorities and researchers continue to work collaboratively to address the complex dynamics of CWD and protect the long-term health of deer ecosystems.

Species Affected by Chronic Wasting Disease (CWD)

Chronic Wasting Disease (CWD) is a transmissible spongiform encephalopathy that affects several species within the deer family, raising concerns about the ecological and conservation implications.

1. White-Tailed Deer (Odocoileus virginianus): White-tailed deer are highly susceptible to CWD, and infections have been reported in various regions where the disease is prevalent. Their widespread distribution and importance in ecosystems make them a key species of concern.

2. Mule Deer (Odocoileus hemionus): Mule deer are also significantly affected by CWD. The disease can impact mule deer populations, leading to changes in behaviour, population dynamics, and ecological interactions.

3. Elk (Cervus): Elk are known to contract and spread CWD, adding to the complexity of disease management. Given the economic and

cultural significance of elk in some regions, addressing CWD in this species is crucial for both wildlife and human interests.

4. Moose (Alces): While less commonly reported than in other deer species, moose can also be affected by CWD. Understanding the occurrence and impact of the disease in moose populations is essential for holistic wildlife management.

The diverse susceptibility of these species contributes to the challenges associated with CWD management, requiring tailored strategies for each affected population. Monitoring and research efforts aim to track the prevalence of CWD in these species, identify factors influencing transmission, and implement measures to mitigate the impact on both wildlife and ecosystems. Controlling the spread of CWD among these susceptible species is crucial for maintaining the health and balance of deer populations and the ecosystems they inhabit.

Geographical Distribution of Chronic Wasting Disease (CWD)

Chronic Wasting Disease (CWD) has exhibited a notable geographical distribution, impacting wildlife populations across different regions and continents. Understanding the spread of CWD is crucial for implementing effective management strategies and preventing further expansion of the disease.

1. North America: CWD was initially identified in mule deer in Colorado in the late 1960s and has since spread to various regions in North America. It affects both white-tailed and mule deer populations, as well as elk and moose. The disease has been reported in several U.S. states and Canadian provinces, creating challenges for wildlife conservation and management efforts.

2. South Korea: CWD has also been identified in South Korea, raising concerns about the potential global spread of the disease. Cases in South Korea highlight the need for international

collaboration in monitoring and addressing CWD.

3. Europe: While less widespread, isolated cases of CWD have been reported in Europe. These occurrences emphasize the importance of continued surveillance and research to understand the factors influencing the disease's spread across continents.

4. Global Concerns: The global movement of wildlife, whether natural or human-mediated, poses challenges in containing CWD. The disease's potential to impact different deer species and its resistance to environmental degradation contribute to its persistence and spread across diverse ecosystems.

Efforts to manage CWD involve not only monitoring and controlling the disease within affected regions but also implementing measures to prevent its introduction into new areas. Collaborative research and international cooperation are crucial for developing a comprehensive understanding of CWD's geographical distribution and formulating strategies to safeguard wildlife and prevent potential transmission to other species, including humans.

Clinical Symptoms of Chronic Wasting Disease (CWD) in Deer

Chronic Wasting Disease (CWD) manifests a distinctive set of clinical symptoms in infected deer, providing critical indicators for diagnosis and management.

1. Progressive Weight Loss: One of the hallmark signs of CWD in deer is a gradual and progressive weight loss. Infected individuals experience a wasting syndrome, leading to a noticeable decline in body condition over time.

2. Altered Behaviour: CWD-infected deer often exhibit significant changes in behaviour. This may include increased aggression, disorientation, repetitive movements, and reduced responsiveness to external stimuli. These behavioural alterations are indicative of the neurological damage caused by the accumulation of misfolded prion proteins in the brain.

3. Excessive Salivation (Drooling): Deer affected by CWD may display increased

salivation or drooling. This symptom is a result of impaired motor function and coordination, affecting the deer's ability to swallow normally.

4. Physical Debilitation: As the disease progresses, deer experience physical debilitation, including weakness, difficulty standing, and an unsteady gait. These motor impairments are a direct consequence of the damage to the nervous system caused by the presence of abnormal prion proteins.

5. Polydipsia (Increased Thirst): CWD-infected deer may exhibit increased thirst, a condition known as polydipsia. This excessive drinking is linked to the impact of the disease on neurological functions, disrupting normal physiological regulation.

Observing and recognizing these clinical symptoms is crucial for early detection and intervention efforts. Identifying CWD-infected individuals allows for targeted management strategies, including the removal of affected individuals from populations to prevent further spread. Additionally, understanding the clinical presentation in deer contributes to ongoing research aimed at unravelling the complexities of CWD and developing strategies for its control and prevention in wildlife populations.

Chapter 4

Causative Agents of Chronic Wasting Disease (CWD): Prions

The causative agents of Chronic Wasting Disease (CWD) are abnormal proteins known as prions. Prions are unique in their ability to trigger a chain reaction of misfolding in normal, healthy proteins, leading to the formation of insoluble aggregates. In the case of CWD, these misfolded prions accumulate in the brain, causing severe neurological damage.

1. Nature of Prions: Prions are unconventional infectious agents primarily composed of misfolded versions of a normal cellular protein called PrP (prion protein). The altered conformation of PrP in prions is remarkably stable and resistant to standard sterilization methods.

2. Accumulation in the Brain: The central event in CWD pathology is the accumulation of misfolded prions in the brain tissue of infected

deer. This accumulation disrupts normal cellular function, leading to the characteristic spongiform degeneration observed in affected individuals.

3. Transmission Mechanisms: Prions are transmitted through various mechanisms, including direct contact between infected and susceptible individuals, ingestion of contaminated material, and environmental exposure. The robust nature of prions allows them to persist in the environment, contributing to ongoing transmission.

4. Role in Transmissible Spongiform Encephalopathies (TSE): Prions are central to the development of Transmissible Spongiform Encephalopathies (TSE), a group of neurodegenerative diseases that includes CWD. The misfolding of prion proteins triggers a cascade effect, inducing neighboring proteins to adopt the abnormal conformation, leading to the spread of pathological changes throughout the brain.

5. Challenges in Detection: Detecting prions poses significant challenges due to their resistance to traditional disinfection methods and the lack of nucleic acid (DNA or RNA) as a target for conventional diagnostic techniques. Specialized assays and techniques are required for the accurate detection of prions.

Understanding the role of prions as the causative agents of CWD is fundamental to developing effective strategies for disease management, preventing further transmission, and safeguarding both wildlife populations and potential human health risks associated with these infectious proteins. Ongoing research continues to explore the intricacies of prion biology and their implications for CWD and related neurodegenerative diseases.

Prions: The Culprit in Chronic Wasting Disease (CWD)

Prions, misfolded proteins with an unusual ability to self-propagate, stand at the core of the

development and progression of Chronic
Wasting Disease (CWD) in deer.

1. Misfolded Protein Cascades: The prion
protein (PrP), normally present in a harmless
cellular form, undergoes a spontaneous and
pathological misfolding process in CWD.
Misfolded prions induce a chain reaction,
causing neighboring healthy PrP proteins to
adopt the same abnormal conformation.

2. Accumulation in the Brain: The misfolded
prion proteins accumulate in the brain tissues of
infected deer, particularly in the central nervous
system. This accumulation disrupts normal
cellular functions, leading to the characteristic
spongiform degeneration observed in affected
individuals.

3. Neurological Damage: The accumulation of
misfolded prions results in severe neurological
damage, affecting the behaviour, motor
functions, and overall health of infected deer.
This progressive degeneration is irreversible
and ultimately fatal.

4. Resistance to Degradation: Prions exhibit remarkable resistance to standard disinfection methods. Their ability to persist in the environment poses challenges for controlling the spread of CWD, as contaminated materials and surfaces can serve as reservoirs for transmission.

5. Transmissible Spongiform Encephalopathy (TSE): CWD belongs to the family of Transmissible Spongiform Encephalopathies (TSE), which includes similar neurodegenerative diseases in other species, such as Creutzfeldt-Jakob Disease (CJD) in humans and Bovine Spongiform Encephalopathy (BSE) in cattle. The commonality across TSEs lies in the misfolding of prion proteins.

Link Between Prions and Transmissible Spongiform Encephalopathy (TSE)

The connection between prions and Transmissible Spongiform Encephalopathy (TSE) forms the foundation of understanding the pathogenesis of diseases like Chronic Wasting Disease (CWD) in deer.

1. Prions as Abnormal Proteins: Prions are abnormal isoforms of a normal cellular protein called the prion protein (PrP). In their misfolded state, prions have the ability to induce healthy, properly folded PrP proteins to undergo the same pathological misfolding.

2. Propagation of Misfolding: The link between prions and TSE lies in the unique ability of misfolded prions to propagate their abnormal conformation. This self-propagation occurs through a templating process, where misfolded prions induce neighbouring normal proteins to adopt the pathological conformation.

3. Accumulation in the Brain: In TSEs like CWD, misfolded prions accumulate in the brain tissue, particularly in the central nervous system. The accumulation disrupts normal cellular function and leads to the distinctive

spongiform degeneration observed in affected individuals.

4. Neurological Consequences: The misfolding and accumulation of prions result in severe neurological damage, causing behavioural changes, motor dysfunction, and, ultimately, the death of the infected individual. This common pathway of neurodegeneration is a defining feature of TSEs.

5. Cross-Species Transmission: The link between prions and TSEs extends beyond deer, encompassing various species. Cross-species transmission is a concern, as evidenced by cases like Bovine Spongiform Encephalopathy (BSE) in cattle, Creutzfeldt-Jakob Disease (CJD) in humans, and Scrapie in sheep.

Understanding the link between prions and TSE is critical for unravelling the complexities of these diseases. Research aims to elucidate the mechanisms underlying prion misfolding, transmission dynamics, and potential avenues for therapeutic interventions. The shared pathogenic processes across TSEs emphasise the importance of comprehensive strategies for disease management and prevention across different species, including wildlife and livestock.

Chapter 5

Epidemiology and Spread of Chronic Wasting Disease (CWD)

Understanding the epidemiology and spread of Chronic Wasting Disease (CWD) is crucial for implementing effective management strategies and mitigating the impact of this transmissible spongiform encephalopathy on deer populations and ecosystems.

1. Factors Influencing Disease Spread:
   - Direct Contact: CWD is primarily spread through direct contact between infected and susceptible individuals. This can occur through social interactions, mating, and shared environments.
   - Contaminated Environment: Contaminated environments, including soil and vegetation, play a significant role in disease transmission. Deer may contract CWD by ingesting prion-contaminated material, perpetuating the spread within ecosystems.

- Animal Movements: The movement of deer, whether natural or human-mediated, contributes to the geographical dissemination of CWD. Infected individuals can introduce the disease to new areas, impacting previously unaffected populations.

2. Surveillance and Monitoring:
   - Early Detection: Robust surveillance programs are essential for the early detection of CWD cases. Monitoring involves testing samples from hunted or culled deer, as well as implementing targeted surveillance in regions at risk.
   - **Wildlife Management:** Surveillance data informs wildlife management strategies, allowing authorities to implement measures such as population control, targeted removal of infected individuals, and other interventions to limit the spread of CWD.
   - Research Initiatives: Ongoing research focuses on understanding the dynamics of CWD transmission, identifying risk factors, and developing improved diagnostic tools. This research is crucial for refining strategies to manage and control the disease.

3. International Collaboration:

- Global Movement of Wildlife: The global movement of wildlife, both natural and human-mediated, necessitates international collaboration in monitoring and addressing CWD. Cooperation among countries and regions is vital for sharing information, coordinating research efforts, and implementing consistent strategies to prevent cross-border transmission.

- Harmonised Regulations: Developing harmonised regulations and guidelines for CWD management facilitates a unified approach to control measures. Shared knowledge and best practices enhance the collective ability to address the challenges posed by this disease.

4. Public Awareness and Education:

- Hunter Outreach: Public awareness campaigns targeted at hunters and the general public are essential for fostering responsible practices. Hunters play a crucial role in disease management, and educating them about CWD transmission dynamics and prevention measures is key.

  - Biosecurity Measures: Implementing biosecurity measures, such as proper disposal of carcasses and hygiene practices, contributes to minimising the risk of CWD transmission.

In summary, a comprehensive understanding of the epidemiology and spread of CWD is fundamental for devising effective and sustainable strategies. Surveillance, research, international collaboration, and public engagement are integral components of a holistic approach to managing and mitigating the impact of Chronic Wasting Disease.

Factors Influencing the Spread of Chronic Wasting Disease (CWD)

The transmission dynamics of Chronic Wasting Disease (CWD) are influenced by various factors, contributing to the spread of this transmissible spongiform encephalopathy within deer populations.

1. Direct Contact:

- Social Interactions: CWD can spread through direct contact between infected and susceptible individuals during social interactions, including grooming, mating, and communal activities.

- Overlapping Home Ranges: Deer with overlapping home ranges are at a higher risk of direct contact. The territorial behavior of deer may facilitate the transmission of CWD within localized populations.

2. Contaminated Environment:

- Soil and Vegetation: Prions, the causative agents of CWD, can persist in the environment, particularly in soil and vegetation. Deer may contract the disease by ingesting prion-contaminated material, contributing to the environmental reservoir of CWD.

- Water Sources: Contaminated water sources can also play a role in disease transmission, especially in regions where infected deer deposit prions through bodily fluids.

3. Animal Movements:

- Migration Patterns: The natural movement and migration patterns of deer contribute to the geographical spread of CWD. Infected individuals can introduce the disease to new areas, affecting previously unexposed populations.

- Human-Mediated Movement: Human activities, such as the relocation of deer for population management or the transportation of infected carcasses, can facilitate the artificial spread of CWD to new regions.

4. Population Density:

- High Density Areas: Regions with high deer population density are more susceptible to CWD spread due to increased opportunities for direct contact and environmental contamination.

- Aggregated Feeding Sites: Artificially concentrated feeding sites, where deer gather closely, can amplify the risk of disease transmission among individuals.

5. Genetic Susceptibility:

- Genetic Factors: Genetic variations within deer populations may influence susceptibility to CWD. Certain genetic factors may make some individuals more prone to infection, affecting the prevalence and spread of the disease.

6. Age and Sex Distribution:
- Social Behavior: The social behaviour of deer, influenced by age and sex distribution, can impact the spread of CWD. For example, interactions during the mating season may contribute to transmission.

Understanding these factors is essential for developing targeted strategies to manage and control the spread of CWD. Effective surveillance, population management, and public awareness initiatives can be tailored based on the specific influences that drive the transmission dynamics of this concerning wildlife disease.

Surveillance and Monitoring for Chronic Wasting Disease (CWD)

Surveillance and monitoring efforts are critical components of managing and controlling the spread of Chronic Wasting Disease (CWD) within deer populations. These strategies play a key role in early detection, informed decision-making, and the implementation of effective disease management measures.

1. Early Detection:
   - Wildlife Testing Programs: Robust surveillance programs involve the systematic testing of deer populations for CWD. Samples are often collected from hunted or culled deer to identify infected individuals.
   - Targeted Surveillance: In regions where CWD is prevalent or poses a high risk, targeted surveillance focuses on specific populations to identify early cases and understand the disease's prevalence and distribution.

2. Wildlife Management Strategies:

- Data-Informed Decisions: Surveillance data provides critical information for wildlife managers and authorities to make informed decisions. This may include adjusting hunting quotas, implementing population control measures, or initiating targeted interventions in areas with confirmed CWD cases.

- Population Modelling: Surveillance data contributes to population modelling, allowing wildlife managers to assess the impact of CWD on deer populations and develop strategies for sustainable management.

3. Research Initiatives:

- Understanding Transmission Dynamics: Surveillance data supports research initiatives aimed at understanding the transmission dynamics of CWD. This includes investigating factors influencing the spread, identifying potential reservoirs, and assessing genetic and environmental influences.

- Diagnostic Tool Development: Ongoing research aims to improve diagnostic tools for CWD. Advances in testing methodologies enhance the accuracy and efficiency of surveillance efforts.

4. International Collaboration:

- Information Sharing: International collaboration is crucial for sharing surveillance data, research findings, and best practices. This cooperative approach helps create a unified front against the global spread of CWD and other transmissible diseases.

- Harmonized Surveillance Protocols: Standardised surveillance protocols facilitate consistent data collection and reporting, enabling comparisons between regions and enhancing the effectiveness of global disease management.

5. Public Awareness and Engagement:

- Hunter Outreach Programs: Engaging hunters and the public in surveillance efforts is vital. Hunter outreach programs encourage reporting of sick or abnormal-looking deer and promote responsible practices for minimising disease transmission.

- Biosecurity Measures: Public awareness initiatives emphasise biosecurity measures, such as proper carcass disposal and hygiene practices, to reduce the risk of CWD spread during hunting and outdoor activities.

Surveillance and monitoring are dynamic processes that evolve with the changing dynamics of CWD. The integration of data-driven decision-making, research advancements, and international collaboration strengthens the collective effort to manage and mitigate the impact of Chronic Wasting Disease on wildlife and ecosystems.